Does my child have a food allergy?

A pocket guide for parents

Second Edition

Written by a pediatric allergist and mother:
The information you need to know about recognizing
possible food allergies in the children you care for.

Jackie Garrett, MD

ISBN: 9781719881128

DEDICATION

To Bear- We started with *Aquamarine* in separate spaces reaching for the stars. Tigers and youthful indiscretions brought us together. Now, as we call a valley home, three shining stars in our midst, the future seems uncertain for our kind, but together with love we will continue to weather the storms of life.

To my greatest treasures - You make me so proud and I love you fiercely. Let this book remind you that achievements are still possible while passing through the lens of true, kind and necessary.

CONTENTS

PREFACE

Food allergy is an unfortunate health event that happens because of an immune response that can be reproduced with each exposure to a particular food. Food allergies affect approximately 6 million children (8% of children) in the United States alone. This may seem like a small number, but for the families who are affected, the path to diagnosis can be long and filled with unnecessary procedures. Food allergies can present themselves in various ways. It is easy to tell that someone is having a food allergic reaction when they have trouble breathing every time they eat a particular food, whereas, more subtle manifestations of food allergies can be frustrating to diagnose in a timely fashion.

In my day to day practice, I come across families who have had a battery of unnecessary tests to finally reach the correct diagnosis. Others are incorrectly diagnosed with food allergies when they actually have an enzyme deficiency. Some of these children, and their parents, end up malnourished after having their diets restricted. Their parents come in scared that their children cannot eat normally, or lead a normal life, because they are at risk of a reaction. Others are frustrated because these diets are nearly impossible to maintain.

This book is for parents, grandparents and caregivers. This book is a quick guide to help you figure out if your child (or even you) may be having a food allergic reaction. This book has been updated with pictures, an allergy doctor approved example of a food allergy action plan and a FAQ section, which were requests after the first edition.

I have divided this book into chapters by symptom category. With some sections I have included examples, not based on any one patient. They are fictional examples to help you see how subtle food allergic reactions can be initially noticed.

I hope this book helps ease parental fears and public confusion about food allergies. I also hope that it helps to guide your discussion with your primary care provider and allergy and immunology specialist.

This book is not medical advice and is not meant to replace an actual consultation with a licensed, board-certified physician. In the field of food allergy in particular, medical knowledge and practice can change quickly. Please do not use this book as a substitute for professional medical advice.

CHAPTER 1: RASHES

There are three main types of rashes that can be a cause of great concern for parents when they go to see an allergist. They are hives, atopic dermatitis (commonly known as eczema), and contact dermatitis.

SECTION 1: HIVES

What are hives?

Hives are a type of rash that can be an allergic skin reaction to a food. The rash has various appearances, including small to large reddish or pinkish areas with central swelling. They can also look like a fluid filled bubble. Hives are often itchy, but can burn. The rash can at times be described as blotches or welts. Hives can show up in a straight line, merging circles or small bumps that are spread apart. Hives can be part of mild allergic reaction, if only a small amount of skin is involved. For example, a few dots on the face. They can at times be part of a severe allergic reaction, if the rash is spread all over the body, or if it is happening with other symptoms.

When should you consider the possibility of a food allergy:

If your child always develops hives after eating a certain type of food.

Example: This is an example of a child with an egg allergy.

- 1st time eating egg product: 8 month old eats a few bites of pancakes and within seconds develops a few blotches on the face (some reactions can take up to 2 hours).
- 2nd time eating egg product: Same child eats a couple of bites of scrambled eggs and within a few minutes, they again develop blotches. This time there are large welts with blotches on face and neck.

What do you do if your child has hives for first time?

If your child fits any of the examples listed above, please contact your primary care provider for advice during the episodes. If you think your child is having a life threatening reaction or if you have had to use an epinephrine auto injector device, call 911.

After the reaction: Make an appointment to talk to your primary care provider about a referral to a board-certified allergist & immunologist.

What to expect at a visit with allergy doctor:

Procedures:

- Skin prick (scratch) testing tests against possible allergen (cause of reaction), results in 15 minutes.
- Laboratory tests: the doctor will order laboratory testing for IgE that corresponds to the protein content of the particular food that is causing concern.

Paperwork:

- Food allergy action plan to help you and other caregivers treat future reactions in your child.

Follow-up:

- Routine follow-up in 1 to 2 years depending on the age of the child since some food allergies can be outgrown.

SECTION 2: ECZEMA

What is eczema?

Eczema, also known as atopic dermatitis, is a skin condition where one develops repeated, red, itchy rashes. The rash can be flat patches of dry scaling skin. The skin can be rough to touch. For darker skin, the areas where the rash develops frequently may become "hyperpigmented", which means darker than the rest of the skin. Skin affected by eczema can be very dry and sensitive.

When should you consider a food allergy:

36% of children with moderate to severe eczema have a food allergy.

- If it seems like your child's skin is never clear despite changing their bath soap, skin lotion and/or prescribed creams.
- If your child frequently needs high dose steroid creams or ointments to help clear the rash and rash returns as soon as you stopping using these products for the prescribed number of days.
- If the eczema is so bad, that your child needs antibiotics for infections of the rash.
- If it seems like your child has more rash than normal skin.
- If your child is always itching. Sometimes, these kiddos keep waking up in the middle of night with the itching. Some parents report blood on the sheets in the morning because the child scratches so hard.
- If within a few seconds to a couple of hours of eating a particular food, they seem to get a new eczema patch or an old patch becomes red or the itching gets worse.

What to do if you think your child's rash is due to a food:

If you are unsure if a food is involved, please contact your primary care provider for advice. In some cases, you may be advised to try to stop giving your child that type of food only for a couple of weeks. Then, add it back in to see if eczema gets worse again.

Example: This is an example of a child with cow's milk (dairy) allergy.

- 4 month old baby who had some patches of eczema on cheeks and back of neck while mom was breastfeeding.
- Age 5 months, started on cow's milk formula. Eczema spread and now covers belly, back and legs.
- Age 6 months, started yogurt melts and cheese. This baby is now scratching all of the time, not sleeping through the night anymore and seems like their skin is always red with a rash. Pediatrician gives topical steroid cream and it helps the rash a little but the skin never is clear and baby is still itching.
- Age 8 months, parents talk to a friend with a similar story. They try to take all cow's milk out of the diet. They change formula to soy formula. 1 week later, baby seems to scratch less. 2 weeks later skin looks much better. Then, they give baby a bottle of cow's milk formula again and within a few hours, baby is itching all over again. So parents stop cow's milk again.

If you were advised to stop and reintroduce a food and then you have to again stop the food of concern after the reintroduction, please make an appointment to talk to your primary care provider about a referral to a board certified allergist & immunologist.

<u>What to expect at a visit with an allergy doctor:</u>

Procedures:

- Skin prick (scratch) testing tests against possible allergen (food that may be causing reaction), results in 15 minutes.
- Laboratory tests: the doctor will order laboratory testing for IgE that corresponds to the protein content of the particular food that is causing concern.

Paperwork:

- Food allergy action plan to help you and other caregivers treat future reactions in your child.

Follow-up:

- Routine follow-up in 1 to 2 years depending on the age of the child since some food allergies can be outgrown.

SECTION 3: CONTACT DERMATITIS

What is contact dermatitis?

Contact dermatitis can include reactions to fragrances, cleaning products or certain foods. It can look like red bumps on certain parts of the skin that come into contact with the trigger food. It can sometimes be just an area of redness. Citrus fruits, onions and garlic can cause a type of redness that is known as **irritant dermatitis**. With this diagnosis, your child can develop redness only where their skin comes into contact with that type of food.

Example:

- School aged child develops redness on hands whenever they peel an orange. They drink orange juice without a problem.
- A baby develops redness on chin after eating a tomato where the juices dribbled down. This also happens when they eat things with tomato sauce.

What to do:

This diagnosis must be made by your physician. If this type of rash is happening, please call your primary care provider's office for advice on what to do at that time. Then, make an appointment to talk to your primary care provider about the possibility of a referral to a board certified allergist & immunologist.

What to expect at a visit with allergy doctor:

- Contact dermatitis to chemicals is generally diagnosed via patch testing at certain ages.
- With food causing irritant dermatitis, testing is not always necessary. It depends on what happened to your child.

CHAPTER 2: ABDOMINAL "BELLY" PROBLEMS

Abdominal or belly problems can be another sign of a food allergy. Allergic reactions can include repeated belly pain, vomiting, diarrhea and refusing to eat.

SECTION 1: BELLY PAIN

What can belly pain mean:

Belly/abdominal pain that is because of food allergies can be because of different causes. This kind of pain can be a part of a severe food allergic reaction, anaphylaxis, where you need an emergency action plan and medications, including epinephrine autoinjector commonly known as an "EpiPen" (or Auvi-Q). This reaction is called an IgE mediated reaction. This pain can also be a type of reaction where you cannot use epinephrine to treat. Diagnoses like food protein induced enterocolitis (FPIES), as well as eosinophilic esophagitis (EOE) and eosinophilic gastrointestinal disorders (EGID) fall into this category. Other causes of belly pain can be a food intolerance or enzyme deficiency.

When to consider a food allergy:

Food allergic reactions can show up as severe abdominal/belly pain within a few seconds to a couple of hours of eating a certain food. Some children can have the belly pain start several hours after eating a food. At times the child has belly pain every day. This pain can prevent them from taking part in normal activities. In other cases it may be only a slight discomfort.

Examples:

- IgE mediated example of a child with peanut allergy: 2 year old gets a sip of dad's peanut butter smoothie and complains of belly pain within 15 minutes but it goes away in 30 minutes. The following week, this same 2 year old is given a slice of bread with a light layer of peanut butter. After eating the slice, 15 minutes later complains of belly pain, then vomits then develops hives on face.

- Eosinophilic esophagitis example: 13 year old boy starts eating less and complaining of belly pain after he eats. He is able to keep going to school and has otherwise normal activity. After 3 months, he starts complaining that food feels like it is getting stuck so he drinks more and eats less because belly pain is slightly worse. 1 month later, he goes for a regular check-up and has lost 15 pounds. He is referred to a gastroenterologist (Intestinal tract doctor) and has an endoscopy that shows that he has a lot of eosinophils "allergy cells" in his esophagus, the part of the body that allows you to swallow food.

What to do:

If your child fits any of the examples listed above, please contact your primary care provider for advice during the episodes. If you think your child is having a life threatening reaction or if you have had to use an epinephrine auto injector device, call 911.

After the reaction: Make an appointment to talk to your primary care provider about a referral to a board-certified allergist & immunologist.

Depending on the timing of the belly pain, your child may also need to be evaluated by a board certified gastroenterologist.

What to expect at a visit with allergy doctor:

Procedures:

- Skin prick (scratch) testing tests against possible allergen (food that may be cause of reaction), results in 15 minutes.
- Food patch testing for some foods currently in the diet may also be performed, although this kind of test is only helpful when positive.
- Laboratory tests: the doctor may order laboratory testing for IgE that corresponds to the protein content of the particular food that is causing concern.

Paperwork:

- Food allergy action plan to help you and other caregivers treat future reactions in your child.

Follow-up:

- Routine follow-up in 6 months to 2 years depending on the age of the child and the diagnosis since some food allergies can be outgrown.

<u>What to expect at visit with gastroenterology doctor:</u>

Procedures: depends on how bad and how often your child's symptoms are

- Blood draw (labwork)
- Stool (Bowel movement) studies (collecting specimens of your child's stool/bowel movements for testing)
- Endoscopy (possibly) where the child is put to sleep and has a camera that is used to look at the inside of the stomach. Biopsies are taken during this time.
- Colonoscopy (possibly) where the child is put to sleep and has a camera that is used to look at the inside of the colon. Biopsies are taken during this time.

SECTION 2: VOMITING

What can vomiting mean:

Vomiting may be because of a stomach bug, food poisoning or even overeating in children. Vomiting can also be because of different types of food allergies. Vomiting can be a type of IgE mediated food allergy, non IgE mediated food allergy like food protein induced enterocolitis (FPIES), or food intolerance.

When to consider a food allergy:

IgE mediated reaction can be seen in cases of projectile vomiting, that start within a few seconds to a couple of hours after eating a particular food. Another type of reaction, food protein induced enterocolitis (FPIES) can happen several hours after eating a particular food. Your child can also complain of belly pain and then get diarrhea along with the vomiting. At times, these vomiting episodes are so severe that a child may need hospital care for intravenous (IV) fluid rehydration.

The following are some examples of food allergic reactions.

- IgE mediated to peanut: 2 year old gets a sip of dad's peanut butter smoothie and develops a few red spots (hives) on chin after15 minutes, but then hives go away on their own within 30 minutes. The following week, this same child is given a slice of bread with a light layer of peanut butter on it. After eating two bites of the bread, the child begins to vomit a large amount continuously for about 15 minutes.

- Food protein induced enterocolitis (FPIES) to rice: 4 month old starts rice cereal. 1st day takes only a few spoonfuls. 4 hours later, develops vomiting and has repeated episodes every 20 minutes for about 1 hour. 8 hours later develops diarrhea. The next day, he wakes up completely fine. Parents chalk it up to a 24 hour stomach bug. 2 weeks later, they try rice cereal again. Again, he only eats a few spoonfuls and 4 hours later develops vomiting but this time there is no break for more than1 hour. Because it is the middle of the night, parents take baby to hospital for evaluation and baby receives IV fluids and a medication to stop vomiting. Baby was discharged home with diagnosis of stomach bug. 2 weeks later, they try rice cereal again. This time he eats half a small bowl. 4 hours later develops vomiting but this time it keeps going and baby becomes lethargic. The parents call 911 and baby is taken to hospital where he receives IV fluids and a medication to stop vomiting. He is kept in hospital for 2 days because he keeps vomiting with diarrhea. Baby was discharged with diagnosis of FPIES.

What to do:

 If your child fits the examples listed above, then please contact your primary care provider for advice during the episodes. If you think your child is having a life threatening reaction or if you have had to use an epinephrine auto injector device, call 911.

After the reaction: Make an appointment to talk to your primary care provider about a referral to a board-certified allergist & immunologist.

Depending on your child's story, you may also need to be seen by a board certified gastroenterologist.

What to expect at visit with allergy doctor:

Procedures:

- Skin prick (scratch) testing tests against possible allergen (food causing reaction), results in 15 minutes.
- Food patch testing for some foods currently in the diet may also be performed, although it is only helpful when this test is positive.
- Laboratory tests: the doctor may order laboratory testing for IgE that corresponds to the protein content of the particular food that is causing concern.

Paperwork:

- Food allergy action plan to help you and other caregivers treat future reactions in your child.

Follow-up:

- Routine follow-up in 1 to 2 years depending on the age of the child since some food allergies can be outgrown.

SECTION 3: DIARRHEA

What can diarrhea mean:

Like abdominal/belly pain and vomiting, diarrhea can be seen in various circumstances tied to food allergies. Diarrhea can be a type of IgE mediated food allergy, a non IgE mediated food allergy, like food protein induced enterocolitis (FPIES), or food intolerance.

When to consider a food allergy:

With IgE mediated reactions, diarrhea starts within a few seconds to a couple of hours after eating a particular food. With non-IgE mediated reactions like food protein induced enterocolitis (FPIES), diarrhea can happen several hours after eating a particular food and can be accompanied by abdominal pain and vomiting. At times these episodes are so severe that a child may need hospital care for IV fluid rehydration. Some children may experience episodes of daily diarrhea with no normal bowel movements.

The following are some examples of food allergic reactions.

- IgE mediated allergy to cow's milk (Dairy): 1 year old gets a bite of big brother's grilled cheese sandwich and develops a few red spots (hives) on chin after 5 minutes. They go away in 30 minutes on their own. The following week, this same child is given a handful of yogurt melts. 15 minutes after 5 melts, child complains of belly pain, then vomits, develops diarrhea and becomes pale.

- Food protein induced enterocolitis, FPIES to oat: 4 month old starts oatmeal cereal. 1st day takes only one spoonful. 4 hours later, develops vomiting for 1 hour. 8 hours later baby develops diarrhea. By the next day the child wakes up completely fine. Parents chalk it up to a stomach bug. 2 weeks later, they try steel cut oatmeal. This time the baby eats 1/2 of a serving. Again 4 hours later develops vomiting and 8 hours later diarrhea, but this time diarrhea keeps

going through the night into midday and the baby is becoming
listless. Baby is taken to hospital by ambulance for evaluation and
receives IV fluids for rehydration. Baby is hospitalized for 3 days.

What to do:

If your child fits the examples listed above, contact your primary care
provider office for advice during the episodes. If you think your child is
having a life threatening reaction or if you have had to use an epinephrine
auto injector device, call 911.

After the reaction: Make an appointment to talk to your primary care
provider about a referral to a board-certified allergist & immunologist.
Depending on the symptoms, your child may also need to be evaluated by a
board certified gastroenterologist.

What to expect at visit with allergy doctor:

Procedures:

- Skin prick (scratch) testing tests against possible allergen (food
  causing reaction), results in 15 minutes.
- Food patch testing for some foods currently in the diet may also be
  performed, although this test is only helpful when positive.
- Laboratory tests: the doctor may order laboratory testing for IgE
  that corresponds to the protein content of the particular food that
  is causing concern.

Paperwork:

- Food allergy action plan to help you and other caregivers treat
  future reactions in your child.

Follow-up:

- Routine follow-up in 1 to 2 years depending on the age of the child since some food allergies can be outgrown.

What to expect at visit with gastroenterology doctor:

Procedures: depends on how bad and how often your child's symptoms are

- Blood draw (labwork)
- Stool (Bowel movement) studies (collecting specimens of your child's stool/bowel movements for testing)
- Endoscopy (possibly) where the child is put to sleep and has a camera that is used to look at the inside of the stomach and take biopsies at the same time.
- Colonoscopy (possibly) where the child is put to sleep and has a camera that is used to look at the inside of the colon and take biopsies at the same time.

SECTION 4: CONSTIPATION

What can constipation mean:

Depending on the age of the child when constipation starts, there can be a variety of causes. Diet is a common cause. However, for older children, there can be acquired causes, or new medical problems where constipation can happen. There are some medical conditions, for example Celiac disease, where certain foods can trigger constipation. However, with these medical conditions, standard food allergy skin testing or food allergy (IgE) blood testing cannot be used for diagnosis. These tests are not helpful and may confuse the picture leading to a delay in diagnosis.

What to do:

If your child has constipation, then please make an appointment to talk to your primary care provider about how to treat constipation. If this is not helpful and constipation persists, then your child may be referred to a board certified gastroenterologist for further evaluation.

SECTION 5: REFUSING TO EAT

What can refusing to eat mean:

Anyone who takes care of a young child will tell you that refusing to eat is usually a normal behavior. How much and what they will eat can vary from day to day. However, sometimes this behavior can be a result of a food allergy. It can be a type of IgE mediated food allergy or non IgE mediated food allergy like eosinophilic esophagitis. You should suspect a food allergy if your child always refuses to eat only one type of food, for example fish, in any form prepared.

When to consider a food allergy:

These are examples of food allergic causes of children refusing to eat.

- o   Child with IgE mediated soy allergy: 14 months old is offered soy yogurt. Baby takes one spoonful, immediately spits it out and refuses to eat anymore. 2 weeks later, parents tried a different flavor of soy yogurt with same outcome. 1 month later, mom gives a smoothie made with soymilk. Child drinks 1 ounce and develops hives all over body.

- o   Eosinophilic esophagitis: 8 year old girl who has always been small for her age is refusing to eat very much and she says it is because her belly hurts. She says that the pain is worse when she eats french fries, mashed potatoes and anything with cow's milk (dairy). Parents eliminate all dairy products and she gets better. She is seen by gastrointestinal doctor who does an endoscopy and results are not normal. They then stop her from eating any potato product. 3 months later the endoscopy was repeated and is now normal.

<u>**What to do:**</u>

If your child is refusing foods, then you should make an appointment to talk to your primary care provider to see if there is a reason for concern. Your child may be referred to a board certified gastroenterologist and/or allergist & immunologist.

<u>**What to expect at visit with allergy doctor:**</u>

Procedures:

- Skin prick (scratch) testing tests against possible allergen (food that may be cause of problem), results in 15 minutes.
- Food patch testing for foods currently in the diet may also be performed, although it is only helpful when positive.
- Laboratory tests: the doctor may order laboratory testing for IgE that corresponds to the protein content of the particular food that is causing concern.

Paperwork:

- Food allergy action plan to help you and other caregivers treat future reactions in your child.

Follow-up:

- Routine follow-up in 1 to 2 years depending on the age of the child since some food allergies can be outgrown.

<u>**What to expect at visit with gastroenterology doctor:**</u>

Procedures: depends on how bad and how often your child's symptoms are

- Blood draw (labwork)
- Stool (Bowel movement) studies (collecting specimens of your child's stool/bowel movements for testing)

- Endoscopy (possibly) where the child is put to sleep and has a camera that is used to look at the inside of the stomach. Biopsies are taken at the same time
- Colonoscopy (possibly) where the child is put to sleep and has a camera that is used to look at the inside of the colon and take biopsies at the same time.

CHAPTER 3: NOSE AND BREATHING PROBLEMS

If someone told you they had breathing problems after eating a food, you might think that it is related to a food allergy. However, sometimes in the moment, or if symptoms are not that severe, individuals dismiss small occurrences, until they think back on them, or when similar episodes keep occurring at a later point in time.

SECTION 1: SNEEZING

<u>When could sneezing mean food allergy</u>:

If your child always sneezes after eating a particular food, even when they are otherwise well.

Example of a food allergy to shellfish:

16 year old goes out to eat. Parents order a shrimp cocktail appetizer. She eats 1 shrimp only and begins sneezing. After 30 minutes it goes away. She does not eat any shellfish for a bit. 3 months later, she goes to a clam bake and eats a few grilled shrimp. She immediately starts sneezing, this time it lasts 45 minutes. She feels like her throat is sore with mucous and so she leaves. She feels better by the next day. 1 week later, she eats a few spoonfuls of clam chowder, she begins coughing then she develops hives. Parents calls her doctor's office for advice on what to do. They treat her and schedule a follow-up with her doctor because they are worried she has developed a shellfish allergy.

<u>What to do</u>:

 If your child fits any part of the example listed above, then please contact your primary care provider for advice during the episode. If you think your child is having a life threatening reaction or if you have had to use an epinephrine auto injector device, call 911.

After the reaction: Make an appointment to talk to your primary care provider about a referral to a board-certified allergist & immunologist.

<u>**What to expect at visit with allergy doctor:**</u>

Procedures:

- Skin prick (scratch) testing tests against possible allergen (food that may be cause of reaction), results in 15 minutes.
- Laboratory tests: the doctor may order laboratory testing for IgE that corresponds to the protein content of the particular food that is causing concern.

Paperwork:

- Food allergy action plan to help you and other caregivers treat future reactions in your child.

Follow-up:

- Routine follow-up in 1 to 2 years depending on the age of the child since some food allergies can be outgrown.

SECTION 2: CONGESTION/STUFFY NOSE

<u>When could stuffy nose mean food allergy</u>:

A stuffy nose in a child is often due to illness, like a cold. If your child has allergies to their environment, it can be due to indoor and outdoor allergens like pollen or animal allergies. In some cases, it can also be because of a food allergen.

<u>When to consider food allergy</u>:

If your child always becomes congested after eating a particular food, even when they are otherwise well.

Example of food allergy to fish:

8 year old goes out to eat with family. Dad orders fish and chips. He tastes a bite of Dad's fish and begins sneezing and feels stuffy. By the next day, it goes away. He does not eat any fish until 3 months later when they go out to eat again. This time family orders salmon patties as appetizer. He takes a few bites of a patty, complains nose is very stuffy, then he begins coughing and then develops hives. Parents take him immediately to emergency room. Doctors and parents are concerned that he has developed a fish allergy.

<u>What to do:</u>

If your child fits the example listed above, then you should contact your primary care provider for advice. If you think your child is having a life threatening reaction or if you have had to use an epinephrine auto injector device, call 911.

After the reaction: Make an appointment to talk to your primary care provider about a referral to a board-certified allergist & immunologist.

What to expect at visit with allergy doctor:

Procedures:

- Skin prick (scratch) testing tests against possible allergen (food that may be causing the reaction), results in 15 minutes.
- Laboratory tests: the doctor will order laboratory testing for IgE that corresponds to the protein content of the particular food that is causing concern.

Paperwork:

- Food allergy action plan to help you and other caregivers treat future reactions in your child.

Follow-up:

- Routine follow-up in 1 to 2 years depending on the age of the child since some food allergies can be outgrown.

SECTION 3 : COUGH

What could a cough mean:

Coughing is a way that our body helps us to clear our airways. We cough if we inhale a large amount of smoke. We cough if we start choking on a drink or food. We cough when we are sick and need to get the mucous out of our chest. Some of us cough because we are having an allergic reaction to food.

When to consider food allergy:

If your child always coughs after eating a particular food, even when they are otherwise well.

Example of child with food allergy to tree nuts:

10 year old eats a mini brownie with crushed walnuts and begins coughing. He drinks water and in an hour cough has stopped. 1 month later, he eats a banana nut muffin. He begins coughing, gasping for air and turns blue. 911 is called and he receives epinephrine autoinjector by EMS and all symptoms go away.   He is taken to emergency room for further treatment. Parents make an appointment with pediatrician because they are concerned that he has developed a tree nut allergy.

What to do:

 If your child fits the example listed above, then you should contact your primary care provider for advice. If you think your child is having a life threatening reaction or if you have had to use an epinephrine auto injector device, call 911.

After the reaction: Make an appointment to talk to your primary care provider about a referral to a board-certified allergist & immunologist.

What to expect at a visit with an allergy doctor:

Procedures:

- Skin prick (scratch) testing tests against possible allergen (food that may be causing the reaction), results in 15 minutes.
- Laboratory tests: the doctor will order laboratory testing for IgE that corresponds to the protein content of the particular food that is causing concern.

Paperwork:

- Food allergy action plan to help you and other caregivers treat future reactions in your child.

Follow-up:

- Routine follow-up in 1 to 2 years depending on the age of the child since some food allergies can be outgrown.

CHAPTER 4: OTHER PROBLEMS

This chapter focuses on other symptoms that parents are worried may be due to food allergies.

SECTION 1: POOR WEIGHT GAIN OR POOR GROWTH

Part of the wonder of having children is watching them grow. Growth problems may present as a child who was growing well and is no longer staying on their growth curve for weight and/or height. Growth problems can also show up in babies or children who have difficulty gaining weight. At times, these problems also come with food refusal, abdominal/belly pain or even abnormal stools (constipation/diarrhea). Causes can vary from gene defects like cystic fibrosis, autoimmune disorders like thyroid disease or celiac disease, and yes, at times food allergies. This is not a comprehensive list of all possible causes, but it may help as a reference for some common problems you might encounter.

<u>When to consider a food allergy</u>:

Some food allergic diagnoses like eosinophilic esophagitis and eosinophilic gastroenteritis can accompany growth problems or even malnutrition. If your child is also having food refusal, complaints of belly pain or changes in bowel movements, these diagnoses can be considered.

The following are examples of causes of growth problems.

- o Eosinophilic esophagitis: 8 year old boy starts eating less and complaining of belly pain after he eats. He is able to keep going to school and has normal activity. After 3 months, he starts complaining that food feels like it is getting stuck so he drinks more and eats less because belly pain is slightly worse. It takes him an hour to finish dinner every night. 3 months later, he goes for a regular check-up and he has lost 10 pounds. The pediatrician orders bloodwork and they are normal. He is then referred to a gastroenterologist and has an endoscopy that shows that he has a lot of eosinophils "allergy cells" in his esophagus, the part of the body that allows you to swallow food.

o   Eosinophilic gastroenteritis: 7 year old girl starts eating less and complaining of belly pain after she eats. After 1 month, she tells parents that her bowel movements have changed and they are really runny. She is starting to miss school because she has bowel movements multiple times a day. After 2 weeks she is brought to pediatrician and is tested for infections but everything is normal. She eats less and she has bowel movements less often but she continues with belly pain. She is then referred to a gastroenterologist because she has lost 10 pounds. She has an endoscopy and colonoscopy that shows that she has a lot of eosinophils "allergy cells" in her stomach and colon.

<u>What to do if you suspect a food allergy:</u>

Generally, in these cases your primary care provider starts an evaluation with various steps to try. If the evaluation is normal for the typical causes of childhood growth problems and the child continues not to grow well, then you can discuss with your provider if is appropriate to have a referral to a board certified gastroenterologist, along with a board certified allergist & immunologist.

<u>What to expect at visit with gastroenterology doctor:</u>

- Blood draw (labwork)
- Stool studies (collecting specimens of your child's stool/bowel movements for analysis)
- Endoscopy (possibly) where the child is put to sleep and has a camera that is used to look at the inside of the stomach and biopsies are taken.
- Colonoscopy (possibly) where the child is put to sleep and has a camera that is used to look at the inside of the colon. Biopsies are taken at the same time.
- All of these procedures depend on symptom pattern and severity.

<u>**What to expect at a visit with allergy doctor:**</u>

- Skin prick testing at times combined with blood draw for IgE that corresponds to the protein of the specific food that is causing concern.
- Directed food patch testing to foods currently in diet may also be performed. This test is only helpful if results are positive.
- Poor weight gain and poor growth is NOT an IgE mediated food allergy which means that the treatment will not include an emergency action plan, the use of antihistamines or the use of an epinephrine auto-injector.

SECTION 2: HAIR LOSS

Hair loss is not a form of IgE mediated food allergy. There can be many causes including infection, nutritional status, autoimmune diseases or an early onset of exaggerated hair shedding. If your child is suffering from hair loss, food allergy testing (IgE skin prick testing or IgE blood testing) is not appropriate and is an unnecessary procedure. Make an appointment to talk to your primary care provider about an evaluation of hair loss.

CHAPTER 5: CONCLUSION

The number of children being affected by food allergies is increasing. This book is meant to help a parent or caregiver identify symptoms of food allergies and have the child in their life evaluated in a safe, appropriate manner. I hope this book is helpful to you.

Worrying about your child's health is normal. If your child does not fit one of the criteria listed in this book, but you remain concerned, talk to your health care provider.

CHAPTER 6: RESOURCES

The following pages contain examples of food allergy action plan, available epinephrine auto injectors in the U.S. and common websites approved by allergy and immunology doctors

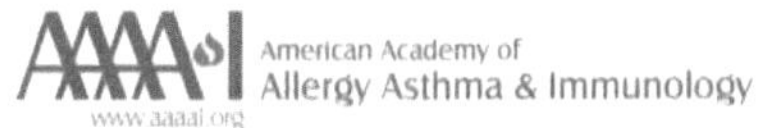

Anaphylaxis Emergency Action Plan

Patient Name: ____ Age: _____________

Allergies: ____

Asthma ☐ Yes *(high risk for severe reaction)*   ☐ No

Additional health problems besides anaphylaxis: ____________________________________

____

Concurrent medications: ____

____

Symptoms of Anaphylaxis

MOUTH	itching, swelling of lips and/or tongue
THROAT*	itching, tightness/closure, hoarseness
SKIN	itching, hives, redness, swelling
GUT	vomiting, diarrhea, cramps
LUNG*	shortness of breath, cough, wheeze
HEART*	weak pulse, dizziness, passing out

Only a few symptoms may be present. Severity of symptoms can change quickly.
**Some symptoms can be life-threatening. ACT FAST!*

Emergency Action Steps - DO NOT HESITATE TO GIVE EPINEPHRINE!

1. Inject epinephrine in thigh using (check one):

☐ **Adrenaclick (0.15 mg)**   ☐ **Adrenaclick (0.3 mg)**

☐ Auvi-Q (0.15 mg)   ☐ Auvi-Q (0.3 mg)

☐ EpiPen Jr (0.15 mg)   ☐ EpiPen (0.3 mg)

Epinephrine Injection, USP Auto-injector- authorized generic
☐ (0.15 mg)   ☐ (0.3 mg)

☐ Other (0.15 mg)   ☐ Other (0.3 mg)

Specify others: ____

IMPORTANT: ASTHMA INHALERS AND/OR ANTIHISTAMINES CAN'T BE DEPENDED ON IN ANAPHYLAXIS.

2. Call 911 or rescue squad (before calling contact)

3. Emergency contact #1: home_________________ work_________________ cell_________________

    Emergency contact #2: home_________________ work_________________ cell_________________

    Emergency contact #3: home_________________ work_________________ cell_________________

Comments: ____

____

____

Doctor's Signature/Date/Phone Number

____

Parent's Signature (for individuals under age 18 yrs)/Date

"Reprinted with permission from the American Academy of Allergy, Asthma & Immunology. Visit AAAAI.org for additional information and updates."

Epinephrine auto-injectors currently available

Auvi Q

- Auvi Q 0.1 mgs (16.5 pounds to 33 pounds)
- Auvi Q 0.15 mgs (33 pounds to 66 pounds)
- Auvi Q 0.3 mgs (66 pounds and up)

Epipen

- Epipen 0.15 mgs (33 pounds to 66 pounds)
- Epipen 0.3 mgs (66 pounds and up)

Generic

- Generic epinephrine auto injectors:
  - Impax generic 0.15 mgs (33 pounds to 66 pounds)
  - Impax generic 0.3 mgs (66 pounds and up)
  - Mylan generic 0.15 mgs (33 pounds to 66 pounds)
  - Mylan generic 0.3 mgs (66 pounds and up)

**The doses and weights above are according to the product manufacturer recommendations. For children, 55 pounds and above, food allergy experts have recommended that the 0.3 mg autoinjector dosage be prescribed to avoid underdosing the child during the reaction.

Useful websites

Allergy and Asthma Network

- Patient centered organization that focuses on outreach, education, advocacy and research.
- Website address- http://www.allergyasthmanetwork.org

American Academy of Asthma, Allergy and Immunology (AAAAI)

- Allows you to find an allergy and immunology doctor nationwide.
- Browse your conditions section
- Website address - https://www.aaaai.org/

American College of Asthma, Allergy and Immunology (ACAAI)

- Allows you to find an allergy and immunology doctor nationwide.
- Multiple sections on allergy symptoms
- Website address - https://www.acaai.org/

American Partnership for Eosinophilic Disorders (APFED)

- Organization dedicated to patients and their families coping with eosinophilic disorders.
- Strives to expand education, create awareness, and support research while promoting advocacy among its members.
- Website address - https://apfed.org/

Asthma and Allergy Foundation of America (AAFA)

- Patient oriented website with information on allergies, advocacy, research programs, education on diagnosis and prevention
- Website address - http://www.aafa.org

Food allergy and anaphylaxis connection team (FAACT)

- Organization goal is to raise awareness for all individuals and families affected by food allergies and life-threatening anaphylaxis.
- Information on responding to food allergy bullying, dealing with workplace issues, or eating out at restaurants
- Website address- https://www.foodallergyawareness.org

Food allergy research and education (FARE)

- Patient oriented website with information on common allergens, advocacy, research programs, education
- Free downloadable Food allergy action plan available in English and Spanish on this website
- Website address - https://www.foodallergy.org

International FPIES Association (I-FPIES)

- Organization that funds research and provides education, support and advocacy for patients and with FPIES (food protein induced enterocolitis syndrome)
- Website address- https://www.fpies.org

Images

Cholinergic hives

Fig. 20-3. From Bonafide C, Whitehorn Brown T. *Urticaria and Angioedema*. From Netter's Pediatrics (pg. 122), by Todd Florin et al., 2011, Philadelphia PA, Elsevier Saunders

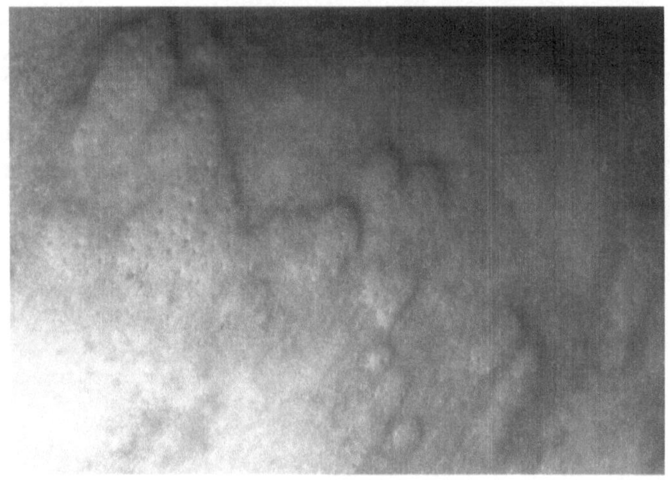

Urticaria (Hives)

Fig. 20-1. From Bonafide C, Whitehorn Brown T. *Urticaria and Angioedema.* From Netter's Pediatrics (pg. 120), by Todd Florin et al., 2011, Philadelphia PA, Elsevier Saunders

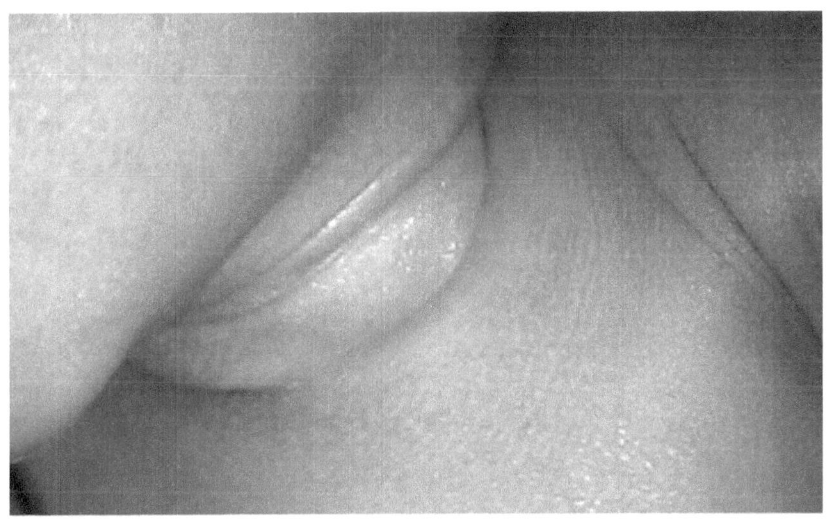

Eczema (atopic dermatitis) with candida

Photo reproduced with parental permission

Eczema (atopic dermatitis)

Photo reproduced with parental permission

FAQ'S

1. What are the most common food allergens?

   Answer: In the U.S. they are Cow's milk (dairy), egg, soy, peanut, tree nuts, fish, shellfish and wheat

2. How old does someone have to be to have a food allergy?

   Answer: Food allergies can happen at any age.

3. If one of my children has a food allergy, will the others be allergic to the same foods?

   Answer: The other children can develop food allergies, not necessarily to the same foods. At this time, there is no good way to predict when and if they will develop food allergies.

4. Should I have my other children tested for food allergies, if their sibling is being diagnosed with one?

   Answer: The current recommendations are that other children should only be tested for food allergies if they are showing symptoms. In the case of peanut, there are other reasons why a baby may be tested before eating the food. Your primary care provider is available to help you with deciding if appropriate to test your baby for peanut allergy before introduction.

5. Can my child grow out of food allergies?

   Answer: Yes, many food allergies are frequently outgrown by late teenage years (Milk, egg, soy are the most common). The likelihood of outgrowing it depends on blood and skin testing. For peanut allergies, there are several ongoing studies/clinical trials on desensitization to help them outgrow these allergies. For tree nuts, there are some allergy practices that are offering desensitization services. These options should be discussed with your allergy and immunology doctor.

6. Did I make my child allergic?

Answer: No!

7. Can I do anything to help my child grow out of food allergies?

Answer: There are certain treatments that are being researched currently. Depending on your child's allergen, there are things that can be done that can help them not have a reaction at a very small dose. This should be discussed with your allergy and immunology doctor.

Glossary of allergy terms

Allergen: The thing that one is allergic to and causes an allergic reaction. It can be a food, animal, pollen, chemical or medication.

Allergy testing types:

<u>Skin prick testing</u>: This is also called a scratch or puncture test. It looks for immediate allergic reactions to specific allergens. The skin is scratched with a device containing the allergen and then results are available in 15 minutes. It can be performed on the forearm or back.

<u>IgE blood testing</u>: Commonly known as RAST testing but that instrument of testing is less favored now and there are better ways to measure IgE. The blood test measures the number of IgE antibodies circulating in the body against a specific allergen. For example, shrimp. This test should be done automatically in combination with skin prick testing because certain types of children, particularly those with eczema, can have positive blood IgE to a certain food and NOT BE ALLERGIC TO A FOOD. This test should be interpreted by a board certified allergist and immunologist to make certain that the right diagnosis is given. Results are generally available in 5-7 days.

<u>Food patch testing</u>: Can be used to diagnose non-IgE mediated food allergy. The data on the usefulness of this test is varied. It can be helpful if positive in the diagnosis of non-IgE mediated food allergies but a negative test does not rule out the diagnosis. It consists of putting small amounts of a single food allergen in a chamber/small disk on the back. It is left on for 48-72 hours.

<u>IgG food testing</u>: AVOID THIS TEST! This type of test is being marketed as a screen for food allergies but that is not a correct interpretation of this test. In all current recognized food allergy studies that look at IgG markers for food, it is actually a marker of increasing TOLERANCE. This means that positive results on this test DOES NOT MEAN that your child is allergic to that food.

IgE mediated food allergy:

The classic food allergy that people think of when they say they have a food allergy. Symptoms occur generally within a few seconds to 2 hours after a specific food exposure. The exception is an allergic reaction to certain meats that occurs 24 hours after ingestion.

Severe symptoms of IgE mediated food allergic reactions are known as Anaphylaxis.

Treatment includes:

- Avoidance of food allergen
- The use of an epinephrine autoinjector (Auvi-Q or EpiPen) for severe reactions, also known as anaphylaxis.
- Epinephrine can be combined with diphenhydramine(common brand name Benadryl), or Cetirizine (common brand name Zyrtec).
- Antihistamines should NEVER replace the use of epinephrine for the management of a severe/anaphylactic food reaction.
- Other medications types can be used depending on severity of reaction.

Diagnosing IgE mediated food allergy: IgE mediated food allergy is diagnosed through skin prick testing (scratch) to the food or food protein that is suspected to have caused symptoms, generally after your child has had a reaction. An exception are the new studies that are suggesting some children should be tested to peanut allergen BEFORE any exposure. (http://www.leapstudy.co.uk/about-leap#.W0T2vdVKgqM).

Since some foods are every similar to one another, if your child reacts to one food in that category, they may have to be tested to other foods in that category. Examples include fish allergy, tree nut allergy and shellfish allergy.

Non IgE mediated food allergy

This kind of food allergy is caused by a reaction involving other cells of the immune system, not IgE antibodies. Some key differences are that these kinds of reactions do NOT appear within a few minutes to a couple of hours after eating the food. They occur several hours after exposure to the food in question. Reactions usually include vomiting and or diarrhea. These children can also have poor weight gain or food refusal.

Specialist Physicians:

<u>Allergy and Immunology</u>:

It is highly recommended that full evaluations for food allergies be performed by a board certified allergist and immunologist. This kind of specialist is a trained medical professional who has done additional training and research, only in allergy and immunology.

This additional training is typically 2-3 years after general practice training. The training involves understanding how the immune system works and how abnormal functioning of the immune system can lead to allergy diagnoses. Because of this training, they are held to practice to the standard of care. That standard is based on current practice parameters on allergic diagnoses, including food allergy. These physicians receive extensive training in interpreting food allergy testing and labs. This minimizes the risk of your child receiving a wrong diagnosis.

<u>Gastroenterology</u>:

These medical professionals are also board certified and are called gastroenterologists. They have done additional training and research, typically 2-3 years after general practice training, only in gastroenterology, hepatology and nutrition.

The training involves understanding how the digestive tract and liver functions. They receive training in nutrition. They are also able to perform endoscopy and colonoscopy and multiple other procedures. Because of this training, they are held to practice to the standard of care that is based on current practice parameters on diseases that affect these parts of the body.